CODE Busters™

QUICK-GUIDE TO CODING AND BILLING COMPLIANCE FOR MEDICAL PRACTICES

Patricia T. Aalseth, RRA, CCS, CPHQ

The author has made every effort to ensure the accuracy of the information herein. However, appropriate information sources should be consulted, especially for new or unfamiliar procedures. It is the responsibility of every practitioner to evaluate the appropriateness of a particular opinion in the context of actual clinical situations and with due considerations to new developments. The author, editors, and the publisher cannot be held responsible for any typographical or other errors found in this book.

Library of Congress Cataloging-in-Publication Data

Aalseth, Patricia T.
CodeBusters' quick guide to coding and billing compliance for medical practices /
Patricia T. Aalseth.
Includes bibliographical references.
ISBN 0-8342-1317-6 (alk. paper)
1. Medicine—Terminology—Code numbers. 2. Health insurance claims—United States—Code numbers. 3. Health insurance claims—United States—Data processing. 4. Medical fees—United States—Data processing. I. Title. II. Title: Quick guide to coding and billing compliance for medical practices. III. Title: Coding and billing compliance for medical practices.
[DNLM: 1. Insurance, Health, Reimbursement—classification handbooks. 2. Patient Credit and Collection—organization & administration handbooks. 3. Fees and Charges—classification handbooks. 4. Financial Management, Hospital—classification handbooks. 5. Practice Management, Medical—economics handbooks. W 49 A112c 1999]
R728.A18   1999
368.38'2'00973—dc21
DNLM/DLC
for Library of Congress
98-43607
CIP

About Aspen Publishers • For more than 35 years, Aspen has been a leading professional publisher in a variety of disciplines. Aspen's vast information resources are available in both print and electronic formats. We are committed to providing the highest quality information available in the most appropriate format for our customers. Visit Aspen's Internet site for more information resources, directories, articles, and a searchable version of Aspen's full catalog, including the most recent publications:
http://www.aspenpublishers.com
Aspen Publishers, Inc. • The hallmark of quality in publishing
Member of the worldwide Wolters Kluwer group.

Editorial Services: Nora Fitzpatrick
Library of Congress Catalog Card Number: 98-43607
ISBN: 0-8342-1317-6

Printed in the United States of America

1 2 3 4 5

Table of Contents

Preface

With health care costs continuing to skyrocket despite the efforts of managed care and other containment programs, third-party payers are scrutinizing every line of every claim for services. When questionable items are identified, their next step is usually a request for copies of your patients' medical records in order to verify that services billed were actually provided. As a physician, whether in a large group or solo practice, you must understand how the coding and billing process works and assure that all official guidelines are being followed by your staff.

This book is a quick reference to the basics of coding for physician services and provides checklists of questions to ask your staff and/or yourself. Also included are suggested resources for additional assistance with coding and billing problems.

Questions in the chapter on patient records (Chapter 2) are vital. There is no point in debating the nuances of coding if the documentation isn't there to begin with. However, good documentation doesn't necessarily mean more documentation. Tips on how to be concise are included.

Thorough use of the checklists will assist you in identifying opportunities for improvement in your coding practices. The information included is the most currently available as of the date of publication; however, the book is not intended as a source of legal advice regarding financial transactions in your business. In particular, should you identify coding errors that may have inappropriately inflated reimbursement already received, it is important that you seek legal guidance.

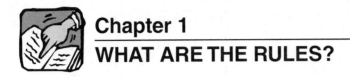

Chapter 1

WHAT ARE THE RULES?

Who is responsible for the accuracy of coding on claims submitted by my office?

Regardless of who actually assigns codes to the services billed, the provider whose name appears on the claim form for physician services is responsible.

The provider's signature block on the HCFA-1500 form, used for submitting claims for physician services, states "I certify that the statements on the reverse apply to this bill and are made a part thereof." On the reverse side of the form appears this statement:

> I certify that the services shown on this form were medically indicated and necessary for the health of this patient and were personally furnished by me or were furnished incident to my professional service by my employee under my immediate personal supervision . . .

If the codes you submit do not match the services documented in the patient's medical record, you may receive reimbursement to which you are not entitled. Another statement of note on the back of the claim form is this:

> Notice: Any person who knowingly files a statement of claim containing any misrepresentation or any false, incomplete or misleading information may be guilty of a criminal act punishable under law and may be subject to civil penalties.

Do not take these statements lightly. Providers have already been prosecuted and convicted under provisions of the federal False Claims Act, which no longer contains a requirement of specific intent to defraud. The word "knowingly" may now include "deliberate ignorance" or "reckless disregard." If your practice has been coding incorrectly over a period of time, resulting in inappropriate reimbursement, this could be considered a pattern of which you should have been aware.

What are the coding rules my staff needs to follow?

Diagnosis Coding

ICD-9-CM

Diagnosis coding is done using ICD-9-CM (*International Classification of Diseases, 9th Edition, Clinical Modification*). In addition to diagnosis codes, ICD-9 contains codes that describe signs, symptoms, problems, history, and other conditions that may be the reason for care. The classification system is maintained and updated by two federal agencies, the National Center for Health Statistics and the Health Care Financing Administration (HCFA).

Official Guidelines

Official guidelines for use of ICD-9 codes are published periodically by these agencies and are used by third-party payers who receive federal funds, such as Medicare, Medicaid, Champus, etc. Many state insurance commissions have also adopted regulations dictating the use of these guidelines for all payers. The section pertaining to physician services is titled "Diagnostic Coding and Reporting Guidelines for Outpatient Services (Hospital-Based and Physician Office)." See Appendix A for current guidelines from the National Center for Health Statistics.

Procedure Coding

General

Coding of procedures and other medical services uses CPT (*Current Procedural Terminology*), published and maintained by the American Medical Association (AMA). HCFA contracts with the AMA to use CPT for the Medicare program in an expanded version, called HCPCS (HCFA Common Procedure Coding System), which also includes alphanumeric codes used to bill for supplies, drugs, and durable medical equipment.

Correct Coding Initiative

In 1996, HCFA adopted its "correct coding initiative," designed to prevent inappropriate unbundling of procedures. Unbundling refers to billing the components of a procedure separately in order to obtain higher reimbursement. An example would be billing for an exploratory laparotomy and another open abdominal procedure performed during the same operative episode when only the latter procedure should be billed. Print and electronic references containing the code combinations considered invalid are widely available.

CPT Evaluation and Management

A significant section of CPT is devoted to evaluation and management (E&M) services, the "visit" codes. These codes are complex, and their definitions have changed several times during the past few years; additional revisions are underway. Documentation guidelines for the visit codes were released by HCFA and the AMA in 1994 and have been updated various times. The codes have been a focus of intensive review by regulatory agencies.

How do I find out about the coding rules for nongovernmental payers?

As you become a provider for various managed care plans, review the contracts to determine if they contain provisions related to coding. Be sure to ask for copies of provider manuals or other references regarding coding and claims submission. Make them available to your staff.

One indication that a payer may have different coding rules is a pattern of claims rejected for coding-related reasons (see Chapter 6 for tips on analyzing payment denials). When a problem is identified, your staff should call the payer to determine whether there is a coding issue. A record of all contacts must be maintained for future reference in case you receive inquiries about changes in coding procedures for that payer. Develop a standard form or database, containing:

❏ name of payer

❏ date of call

❏ number called (national, regional, or local office)

❏ name and title of person contacted

❏ question asked

❏ information received

❏ signature/initials of office staff member making call

Why do I need written policies and procedures for coding and billing?

Written policies and procedures are the best method for assuring that you and your staff are on common ground in your understanding of how coding and billing must be done. They are useful in:

❏ training new staff

❏ assuring that all personnel are using consistent procedures

❏ evaluating staff performance

❏ demonstrating to auditors that organized methods are in place

❏ establishing a framework for regular internal quality reviews of coding and billing practices

Policies and procedures need not be voluminous. A simple statement indicating that current official ICD-9-CM coding guidelines will be followed, with an attached copy of the most recent version, will suffice as a start. Once established, policies and procedures must be treated as living organisms, updated as needed to assure compliance with current regulations and payer policies. Assign responsibility for this to a specific staff member.

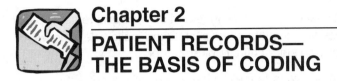

Chapter 2

PATIENT RECORDS— THE BASIS OF CODING

How do I know if my records are good enough to pass an audit?

A patient record audit will look for the same information all payers want:

- ❏ Does the documentation in the record describe services billed?

- ❏ Were the services medically necessary?

- ❏ Were appropriate services provided?

In some instances, the auditor may also contact and interview patients to verify that you provided the services you documented.

Your records are good enough only if you can answer "yes" to all of the above questions.

What can I do to improve my records and documentation?

Sit down with your staff and take a look at a sample of your current records, objectively answering the following questions:

Organization of Record

- ❏ Is the patient's name clearly legible on the outside of the record?

- ❏ Is there a standard filing order to promote easy retrieval of needed information, or are items just filed at random as they come in?

- ❏ Are major database components, such as the history, easy to locate to avoid time-wasting repetitive recording?

- ❏ Can records be located as needed, or do you often have to provide patients care without the record?

- ❏ If your office uses an electronic patient record, is it easy to use and reliable?

❏ If space limitations are causing record storage and retrieval problems, have you implemented a standard policy defining which records may be stored off-site or discarded?

The goal of this review is to make sure you have the correct patient's record available at every visit, in usable condition.

Information Capture on Record

Ask your staff to assemble a complete set of record forms currently used in your practice. Review the forms as a group, answering the following questions:

❏ Are the forms clear and easy to read, or have they been photocopied until they are blurry, crooked, and faint?

❏ Is there a consistent location on each form for the title of the form?

❏ Is there a consistent location on each form for the patient's name and record number, date of birth, or other identifier?

Next, review each form individually, with these issues in mind:

❏ What is the purpose of this form? Determining the purpose will help define the content and format.

❏ Does this current form contain the elements necessary for adequate documentation of services provided?

Example: forms for recording patient history should contain spaces for all items considered part of the history in the E&M services billing code descriptions:

❏ chief complaint (CC)

❏ history of present illness (HPI)

❏ review of systems (ROS)

❏ past/family/social history (PFSH)

See Appendix B, Data Elements for Adequate Documentation, for detailed requirements for specific types of billing codes.

❏ Who will be completing this form? If portions of the form are to be completed by the patient, instructions may be needed.

❏ Does this form use terminology consistent with code descriptions? If an auditor reviews your records, the task will be easier (and the outcome likely more positive) if your documentation is labeled with terms matching the code descriptions.

❏ Is there duplication of documentation on this form and others that could be eliminated?

The goal of this review is to update your record forms, making sure you have only what is necessary to adequately document the services you provide, with no duplication of effort, and to assure that the forms are well-designed and present a professional appearance. Desktop publishing has facilitated in-house form design; the expense of revision is now minimal. If your practice uses an electronic record, the input screens and output formats should be reviewed periodically for clarity and consistency as described above.

Assessing Legibility

Illegibility is a serious problem, not only a billing concern, but also a patient care risk management issue with the potential for misinterpretation of orders, medications, etc. If your patient records are audited, it is not likely that you will be credited with documentation that justifies your billing if the records can't be deciphered.

To face the truth about this issue, try these two tests:

1) Take a record at random and open it to a progress note page. Ask a member of your staff to read it aloud. If they have difficulty, they may be routinely misinterpreting what you write, and may also be incorrectly billing for your services.

2) Ask a staff member to photocopy a page of progress notes from a chart and obliterate the patient's name. Try reading this yourself. If you can't read it, how can you expect that anyone else can?

Improving Legibility

❏ If you have had bad handwriting since the first grade, you are somewhat unlikely to improve it at this point. However, if you feel your writing is dismal because of lack of sufficient space in which to write, make sure you consider this in the review and revision of your office forms. Some individuals with expansive handwriting do fine when given adequate space on a form.

❏ Some portions of the record may be completed by your office staff or even by the patient, as long as you document that you have reviewed the information and confirmed or added to it. This applies to the review of systems (ROS) and the past/family/social history (PFSH) sections.

❏ Another alternative aimed at improved legibility is the use of more forms with printed content outlines, particularly for the physical examination. As long as abnormal or unexpected findings and other pertinent information is recorded in detail, it is acceptable to use check boxes to indicate "negative" or "normal" where appropriate.

❏ Although transcribing office notes adds to expense, it could be worth the cost if an audit occurs. If you choose this method to improve legibility, be sure that 1) the turnaround time is timely; medications and other important items should still be written in the chart for use until the transcribed report is received; and 2) you use a dictation outline containing the elements necessary to justify charges billed.

Other Methods

❏ Make sure your documentation is completed as soon as possible, preferably on the date of the patient visit/encounter. If it is necessary to make a record entry at a later date, be sure to include not only the date of service, but also the actual date the late entry is being made. This is the acceptable method of making late entries.

❏ Include in the entry not only the date of service, but also the time spent, as appropriate. This is imperative when billing time-based services or services where counseling and coordination of care dominate. See Chapters 4 and 5 for details.

❏ Make full use of services provided by hospitals and other facilities where you also see patients. These may include copies of transcribed reports and copies of coding summaries for discharged inpatients. Be sure to include in your records copies of reports from consultants to whom you have referred patients.

❏ Consider the use of flowsheets for repetitive data that needs to be compared over time. Nothing is more frustrating than searching through a chart looking for lab results for the past few months in order to evaluate changes in the patient's condition.

❏ Document in the chart tasks you perform that contribute to the complexity of medical decision making for this patient encounter. These might include:

- consideration of differential diagnoses

- initiation of or changes in treatment

- referrals

- review of lab, radiology, or other diagnostic test results

- review of old records, with relevant findings

- discussion with other physicians

- personal review of images, specimens, etc.

❏ Document anything out of the ordinary. This might include unexpected findings, events that delay or preclude treatment, patient noncompliance, family issues that affect treatment, etc. Should questions arise later, your best defense to "why didn't you?" is to have all the details readily available.

Chapter 3

TRANSLATING THE RECORD
INTO CODES—DIAGNOSIS

The title of this chapter should be taken literally. In many offices, the patient record is "out of the loop" when billing actually takes place. The diagnoses and procedures submitted on claim forms are often taken from a superbill or encounter billing form marked by the physician or nurse, with no verification that the patient record contains justifying documentation. If your practice is audited, the patient record will be the source document. The appropriate time to assure documentation is present is *before* billing takes place.

How do I know which diagnosis codes to use for billing?

The standard claim form (HCFA-1500) has fields for four diagnosis codes. The primary diagnosis should be listed first. This is "the ICD-9-CM code for the diagnosis, condition, problem, or other reason for encounter/ visit shown in the medical record to be chiefly responsible for the services provided" (Appendix A, Section G, Official Guidelines). In addition to the primary diagnosis, you may list additional codes describing coexisting conditions that require or affect treatment or management.

How do I determine which diagnosis is primary?

Code the condition to the highest degree of certainty for that encounter/visit . . . (Appendix A, Section H, Official Guidelines). These examples demonstrate the most important rule of diagnosis coding for physician/outpatient billing:

Chief Complaint

A good place to start would be the chief complaint. This is often documented by office staff; make sure they understand what the concept means. They should not be substituting scheduling terms such as "annual exam" when the patient has a specific complaint or condition to be addressed. Terms such as "routine follow-up" should be replaced with the name of the condition being followed.

In some cases, the chief complaint will end up as the primary diagnosis. If a patient presents with "blood in my urine," and the exam and workup do not produce a definitive cause on the first visit, "hematuria" will be the primary diagnosis for that encounter.

Specific Diagnosis

Often, a more specific diagnosis will be reached after the patient has been examined and the complaints addressed. If the patient is being seen because of cough and fever (chief complaints) and a diagnosis of pneumonia is made, pneumonia is the primary diagnosis.

Why can't I code "rule/out" if that's what I'm doing?

These examples demonstrate the physician billing diagnosis rule of

Do not code diagnoses documented as "probable," "suspected," "questionable," "rule/out" . . . (Appendix A, Section H, Official Guidelines).

The coding of "rule/out" diagnoses as if they already existed is inappropriate because it is not known whether the patient, in fact, has the condition being questioned. Also, coding the "rule/out" condition does not indicate the necessity for diagnostic testing being performed; if you are already certain the patient has the condition, you don't need the testing to make the initial diagnosis.

The process of "ruling out" a condition indicates there are existing signs or symptoms that point toward a likely diagnosis, but prompt "rule/out" testing. What is it that makes you want to rule/out? Use the signs, symptoms, abnormal test results, or other reasons prompting your suspicions as the diagnosis.

What diagnosis do I code if the patient has no complaints?

In addition to "regular" diagnosis and symptom codes, ICD-9-CM also contains a supplemental classification of codes to indicate when:

❏ a person with no current illness is being seen for a specific purpose

❏ a patient with a resolving disease or injury or a chronic condition is being seen for after-care or special therapy

❑ the patient has a history, health status, or other problem that may affect his care, although not in itself a current disease or injury

❑ birth status for newborns

Again, the question to ask is "Why is the patient being seen?" Some of the most common visits of this type are:

❑ school or insurance physicals

❑ long-term anticoagulant use

❑ chemotherapy or dialysis

❑ attention to artificial opening (gastrostomy, colostomy, ileostomy)

❑ elective sterilization

❑ suture removal

❑ fitting and adjustment (includes removal) of catheters

❑ hardware removal

❑ surgery follow-up

❑ fracture follow-up

❑ repeat prescription

❑ contact with communicable disease

❑ supervision of normal pregnancy

❑ screening exams for neoplasms

The codes from this section of ICD-9-CM are known as "V codes" because they are all alphanumeric, starting with a V. Third-party payers are increasingly aware of the appropriate use of these codes and most no longer automatically reject claims with a V code diagnosis. Some HMOs and other managed care plans include preventive medicine benefits such as coverage for an annual routine physical.

If you code for a condition the patient no longer has instead of the appropriate V code for a visit, you are misrepresenting the diagnosis to the payer. Look over the V code section in the ICD-9 book and make sure your staff understands how it is to be used.

How do I know which diagnosis codes will be paid?

The relationship of diagnosis codes to payment is their use in providing medical necessity justification for various procedures. Not only federal payers, but also most other third-party payers have established lists of "covered codes" for individual tests. Example: Medicare requires that, "for coverage to be provided for urinalysis (UA), the patient must have signs or symptoms of a kidney/urinary tract disorder or a condition which is known to affect the kidney/urinary tract." A list of several hundred covered codes accompanies this policy.

Information on which codes are covered can be obtained from your local carrier or from the provider relations department of other payers. The purpose of obtaining this information is to make yourself aware of the instances in which tests will not be covered so you can inform the patients they will be liable for the costs themselves. (Many hospitals and other labs that handle your send-outs have built these edits into their billing software so they know up front when the patient will be responsible for payment.) The purpose of obtaining this information is *not* to make sure you use one of the approved codes every time you order a UA.

Should my staff be using cheat sheets to code?

Cheat sheets (lists of commonly used diagnosis codes) are often used in physician/outpatient offices. If your staff is using one, at least make sure that it is reviewed and updated annually when the official diagnosis coding changes take effect on October 1st. Under no circumstances should your staff be using a cheat sheet that contains headings for various diagnostic tests with only the payable diagnoses for that test listed underneath. This is a definite red flag to an auditor.

Remember that all codes submitted for payment must match the documentation in the patient record. It is more likely this will be the case if your staff codes the record from the coding book or software instead of using the less-specific-but-more-convenient code on the cheat sheet. Lists of codes found on superbills have the same limitations.

What about diagnosis codes related to procedures?

In addition to the four diagnosis codes, the claim form also has fields for six procedure codes. Each procedure can be linked to one of the four diagnosis codes. Let's say you have a patient who is seen with the chief complaint of fever and chills. The workup results in a diagnosis of urinary tract infection (UTI). During the exam, genital warts are identified and destroyed. The primary diagnosis will be the UTI, with the warts as secondary. The procedure code for destruction of warts will be linked on the form to diagnosis number two.

Make sure your staff understands this linking concept. If they do not enter a diagnosis number in the linking column, the payer will assume the procedure is being performed for diagnosis one as a default. This may result in medical necessity denials.

For operative procedures, the postoperative diagnosis should be used as the primary, as the most definitive diagnosis. This may involve waiting for the final pathology report *if* the diagnosis is in question.

Chapter 4
TRANSLATING THE RECORD INTO CODES—PROCEDURES

How do I choose the correct procedure codes?

It is extremely important that you familiarize yourself with the terminology used in codes for the procedures you perform. CPT descriptions are quite detailed, and in some cases, a single word can make the difference between one code and another. Instead of just describing the procedure, CPT sometimes also dictates whether it was performed for a specific indication or diagnosis. Example: there are different codes for vitrectomy and for vitrectomy for repair of retinal detachment. *Read carefully to avoid inappropriate billing.*

CPT descriptions do not always repeat all the words actually contained in the code. Any time you see an indented description, you need to go back up to the unindented description at the top of the section. Read that description until you come to a semicolon. All the words before the semicolon are also intended to be part of the following, indented, codes. Make sure you consider this convention when you are selecting codes.

What kinds of procedures should not be billed?

Medicare and other payers have determined that the following types of procedures should not be billed:

❏ anesthesia administered by the physician performing the medical or surgical procedure

❏ less extensive procedures; if the code descriptions indicate a series of procedures from less to more complex, only bill for the most complex procedure performed from that series

❏ unsuccessful procedures; if a more comprehensive procedure is performed instead, only bill for the latter

❏ procedures integral to surgical procedures, such as skin prep, positioning patient, approach, cultures, irrigation, insertion and removal of drains, simple closure, application of dressings

❑ endoscopic procedure, prior to surgical procedure, for purposes of locating a lesion, establishing landmarks. Note: diagnostic endoscopy that serves as the basis for decision to perform an open procedure *may* be separately billed

❑ procedures described in CPT as "separate procedure" when performed with a more comprehensive procedure

Global Procedures

What is included in a global surgery package?

Most surgical procedures are billed using the concept of a "global" package. The payment for the package covers a defined period of time, usually 0, 10, or 90 days, and includes the surgery, follow-up visits, dressing changes, and surgical supplies.

Some nongovernmental payers have different global periods; it is best to check with the payer to determine what is included.

Is there anything I *can* bill in addition to the global?

Yes. If you do the procedure on the same day you first see a new patient, you can also bill for the visit. For a 90-day global, the visit can be billed even for an established patient if you determined during the visit that the surgery was needed (day of or day prior to surgery).

Also, if you see the patient during the follow-up period but for an unrelated condition, this is separately billable. Any complications are considered to be related and thus not billable, unless another trip to the operating room is required.

In addition, lab tests, X-rays, and other diagnostic testing may be billed.

How do I communicate to the payer that a charge is *not* included in the global?

HCPCS and CPT use two-digit modifiers, appended to the individual procedure codes, to indicate that special circumstances exist. Some of these relate to the global surgical package or to modifications in procedures that may affect payment. These modifiers are currently used by HCFA and also are accepted by many other payers:

❏ –24 Evaluation and management (E&M) service for an unrelated condition during a global surgery period. Example: Patient undergoes total knee replacement on June 1st, then returns to orthopaedist on July 15th for severe pain in elbow. The July office visit must be billed with a –24 modifier and an elbow-related diagnosis in order to be paid.

❏ –25 E&M service on same day as surgery, for unrelated reason. Example: a patient is seen in the office for an ingrown toenail, which is partially excised. During the course of the visit, the provider notes the patient has a severe, productive cough. An exam is performed, X-rays ordered, and substantial effort spent in evaluating what is diagnosed as bronchitis. The nail procedure may be billed, and the visit may also be billed, with a –25 modifier and the bronchitis diagnosis. This modifier is subject to frequent audit; so make sure your record substantiates the significant, separately identifiable E&M service.

❏ –57 Decision for surgery made during E&M visit same day or day before major surgery (90-day globals). Example: Patient is admitted to the hospital with a fracture of the femoral neck. The orthopaedic surgeon examines the patient and determines that open reduction with internal fixation is the appropriate course. The surgery takes place later that day. The surgeon may bill for the surgery and may also use a –57 modifier to bill for the preoperative visit.

❏ –58 Staged procedure. Use on the procedure code for a subsequent procedure that was: a) planned (such as two-stage breast reconstruction); b) required because a less extensive procedure failed (but do not use if there is a complication—see modifier –78 instead); or c) therapeutic procedure following a diagnostic one.

❏ –59 Distinct procedural service. Tells the payer this service was done on the same day, but involved a different operative episode, a different site, a separate lesion, or a separate injury, etc. This modifier is used when the combination of codes you are billing for a given day looks like unbundling, but is not. Example: A patient is admitted through the emergency room with a left shoulder injury, including a penetrating wound in the front and a large hematoma in the back. Coding both the hematoma evacuation and an exploration of the penetrating wound would without the modifier be denied as duplicate billing. Using the –59 modifier on one of the codes to indicate a different site will explain the circumstances. Note: Modifier –59 does not replace –LT, –RT, –24, –25, –78, or –79.

❑ –78 Return to the operating room for complications related to the first surgery during the global period.

❑ –79 Procedure done during global period for unrelated condition. Make sure the diagnosis code for the second procedure is unrelated.

Other HCFA modifiers that may make circumstances clearer are:

❑ –LT left

❑ –RT right

❑ –50 bilateral procedure (do not use if the code definition itself is bilateral)

Unusual Cases

How do I get paid for surgery that takes longer than normal?

❑ –22

It is possible to receive increased reimbursement for a procedure if there are unusual circumstances that cause it to be more extensive than normal. Example: Lysis of abdominal adhesions is considered a normal part of a surgical procedure. However, if you have an obese patient with very extensive adhesions and it takes 30 minutes longer than normal to perform the procedure because of them, you may add a –22 modifier to your surgery code. Be sure to use the diagnosis code for adhesions in addition to the diagnosis code for the condition necessitating surgery. It is also a good idea to submit a copy of the operative report with the unusual circumstances highlighted.

❑ –52 and –53

There are two modifiers, –52 and –53, for reduced services and discontinued procedures, which should be reported as appropriate. Contact the payer for information regarding their acceptance of these modifiers.

How do I submit copies of documentation for unusual cases if I file my claims electronically?

This is important—Making sure your reports get to the person who will determine medical necessity may require extra effort on your part. Using a transmittal form to submit these reports should help. It must contain, at the very least: patient identification, provider identification, date of service, and the procedure codes for which you are providing the information. Contact the payer and determine their procedures for submitting these materials. Keep a copy of the transmittal form in the patient's record so you will know what has been sent and when.

Chapter 5

TRANSLATING THE RECORD INTO CODES—EVALUATION & MANAGEMENT

Evaluation and management (E&M) codes were implemented in 1992 and have since been revised several times. Because of the extremely complex nature of the codes, HCFA and the AMA published documentation guidelines for each type of code. These guidelines have been used in auditing patient records. It is extremely important to be sure you are documenting and billing correctly for these codes as they are a fraud and abuse focus area.

Definitions used in E&M code selection:

New patient: has not received professional services from you or another provider *of the same specialty* in your group during the past three years. When a provider enrolls in Medicare or other payer plans, they are designated as a particular specialty. Problems may result when subspecialists in the same group do not have an "official specialty" and "new patient" claims are denied or downgraded as a result. This has been true on occasion for Pain Medicine, Maternal–Fetal Medicine, and other subspecialties that are often assigned to the more general categories of practice.

Consultation: your opinion or advice regarding a specific problem is requested by another physician. A confirmatory consultation is a "second opinion." Note: Once you complete your initial consult, if you assume responsibility for managing any of the patient's conditions, you are no longer a consultant.

Intra-service time: Office/outpatient: face-to-face. The time the physician spends with the patient and/or family.

Hospital/inpatient: unit/floor time: Time spent on the patient's unit, including face-to-face, plus chart review and documentation and communication with other professionals.

Initial: the first service of that type, per admission. Do not charge for more than one initial service per admission.

How do I choose the correct code based on the documentation in the patient's record?

Answer the following questions. A blank review sheet is found at the end of this chapter, which you can copy for use by your staff in assessing the correct level of care for patient visits.

Did you spend more than 50% of the time you were with the patient and/or family on counseling and/or coordination of care?

An example of adequate documentation for this type of visit would be a case in which the surgeon discusses malignant pathology findings with the patient. The prognosis and various treatment options with their respective risks and benefits would be covered. In the chart note, the total intra-service time is indicated immediately after the date and then the amount of time spent in discussion and the topics of the discussion are documented. Later in the patient's hospital stay, the discussion might be centered on instructions for follow-up, emphasis on compliance with treatment, and arrangements for care such as home health services.

If the time spent on counseling and coordination of care constitutes more than 50% of the total time for that visit, the selection of E&M code may be based on time alone.

This method of assigning an E&M code may only be used with codes for which average times have been established. These include:

Services	Intra-service time definitions				
Office/outpatient—new	10	20	30	45	60
Office/outpatient—established	5	10	15	25	40
Outpatient consult	15	30	40	60	80
Inpatient—initial care	30	50	70		
Inpatient—subsequent care	15	25	35		
Inpatient—initial consultation	20	40	55		
Inpatient—follow-up consult	10	20	30		
Nursing facility—assessments	30	40	50		
Nursing facility—subsequent care	15	25	35		
Home visit—new	20	30	45	60	75
Home visit—established	15	25	40	60	

It is extremely important that your documentation for this type of code assignment include the total time, the time spent on counseling and coordination of care, and what transpired during the visit.

Were your services provided to newborns or to critically ill infants?

E&M services for these patients are coded using *per day* codes based on the location and/or condition of the infant:

Critical: Initial day for critically ill patient
Subsequent day for critically ill, unstable patient
Subsequent day for critically ill, stable patient

Other: Initial history and physical (H&P) for normal newborn in hospital setting
Subsequent day for normal newborn
Initial H&P and discharge of newborn in and out same day
Normal newborn care in other than hospital setting

Did your services involve discharging the patient from this episode of care?

Discharge day management codes are available for Observation, Inpatient, and Nursing Facility sites of service. They include patient exam, discussion, instructions for continuing care, and preparation of discharge record, referral forms, prescriptions, etc. This is another area where it is imperative to document the amount of time spent, as several of these codes are time-dependent. Codes for inpatients or observation patients who are admitted and discharged on the same date are also distinct.

Did you provide critical care?

Patients may receive critical care in any setting; it is the patient's condition and need for intensive services that determine critical care, not their location. Patients requiring critical care are unstable and critically ill or critically injured. Constant physician attendance is required. It need not be continuous throughout a given calendar day; the total time spent for that day is used to assign codes. Constant attendance does not mean the provider is at the bedside, but it does mean that he or she is performing tasks directly related to that individual patient's care. Many services, such as interpretation of blood gases, electrocardiograms, vent management, and vascular catheterization are included in the E&M codes for critical care.

If you have a patient in the unit, document carefully the following for each visit: total time spent and what you did during that time. If you spent less than 30 minutes total for the date, use a "regular" visit code instead of a critical care code. Refer to the excellent examples in the CPT book for calculating assignment of critical care codes.

What can you do when you end up spending too much time with a patient who is having a crisis but doesn't require critical care?

The prolonged services codes can account for this effort. There are face-to-face and non-face-to-face codes, calculated on the amount of time spent *over and above* another time-based code. The non-face-to-face prolonged services codes must be used on a day when there is also face-to-face patient contact, either before or after the prolonged service.

Payers vary greatly in covering this category of services. As with other time-based services, detailed documentation of what you did and how long it took is imperative.

What about procedures for routine physicals and other exams when the patient has no complaints?

❑ Preventive medicine codes, age-based and divided by new/established patient, are used for a visit with this purpose. Included are a comprehensive history and exam, plus ordering lab and other diagnostic procedures, and counseling.

❑ If the purpose of the encounter is specifically for patient education, the preventive medicine counseling codes can be used.

❑ Exams, without ensuing problem management, for administrative purposes such as insurance, workers' compensation, or disability also have separate codes.

Can considerable amounts of time on the telephone, adjusting medications, and giving new orders for other treatments for home health, nursing home, and hospice patients be billed?

Care plan oversight, developed to address this issue, is a "forgotten service" that many physicians do not bill. The key to this billing is, as usual, being able to prove that the required amount of time was spent. An efficient method of tracking this time is a care plan oversight form for each patient receiving these services, filed in a notebook on your desk. It is designed with the days of the month down the left side and the months of the year across the top. Phone calls and other communication regarding these patients is noted in the actual record, as usual, but the number of minutes spent on that day is placed in the appropriate box on the form in the notebook. At the end of the calendar month, your staff can add up the minutes for that month. If the total is more than 15 minutes, you have a billable service. At the end of the calendar year, the form is filed in the patient's record. See the definitions in your CPT book for more details.

What about E&M services that don't fall into any of the categories above? These would include:

❑ No standard times determined:

- Observation care

- Emergency department

- Boarding home

- Confirmatory consults

❑ Services with time standards, but:

- Counseling/coordination of care *not* more than 50% of time spent

In order to correctly assess and assign a level of care for these services, you will need to determine at what level these three key elements are documented: history, exam, and medical decision making.

Medical decision making—how to document it

❑ Did you make differential diagnoses for new problems?

❑ Are existing problems improving, resolving, worsening, etc.?

❑ What treatment was initiated or changed?

❑ What types of data were reviewed; did you obtain old records?

❑ Did you look at films or other data already interpreted by others?

❑ Were referrals made to consultants? Whom and why?

❏ Do your adjectives reflect the true severity of the patient's presenting problems?

❏ What other conditions were present that increase the complexity of your medical decision making?

❏ What types of diagnostic procedures did you order, perform, or schedule?

❏ How will you be managing this patient's conditions; medications, IV fluids, surgical procedures?

Use the audit tool on the next few pages to assess your documentation.

EVALUATION AND MANAGEMENT AUDIT—HISTORY

Mark elements present, count them, and then circle type at right of each area.

History of Present Illness (HPI)

❑ location   Brief = 1–3 elements

❑ quality

❑ severity   Extended = 4 or more elements

❑ duration

❑ timing

❑ context

❑ modifying factors

❑ associated signs /symptoms

Review of Systems (ROS)

❑ constitutional   None = 0 elements

❑ eyes

❑ ENT, mouth   Problem-pertinent = 1 element

❑ cardiovascular

❑ respiratory   Extended = 2–9 elements

❑ gastrointestinal

❑ genitourinary   Complete = 10 or more elements

❑ musculoskeletal   or notation of "all others negative"

❑ skin/breast

❑ neurologic

❑ psychiatric

❑ endocrine

❑ heme/lymph

❑ allergy/immune

Past, Family, and/or Social History (PFSH)

❑ past   None

❑ family   Pertinent = 1 area

❑ social   Complete = 2–3 areas

ASSESSMENT OF HISTORY: From the lists above, circle the appropriate entries for HPI, ROS, and PFSH on the grid below. Find the circle farthest to the left, and draw a line straight down to the type of history.

HPI	Brief	Brief	Extended	Extended
ROS	None	Prob-pert	Extended	Complete
PFSH	None	None	Pertinent	Complete
History	Problem-focused	Expand prob-foc	Detailed	Comprehensive

EVALUATION AND MANAGEMENT AUDIT—EXAM

Mark the elements present, count them, and then circle the type at right. For additional details about what is included in each portion of the physical exam, see Appendix B. This audit tool is intended only for the general multisystem exam. Specialists should contact HCFA for information about the contents of various single-specialty exams.

❑ constitutional
❑ eyes
❑ ENT, mouth
❑ cardiovascular
❑ respiratory
❑ gastrointestinal
❑ genitourinary
❑ musculoskeletal
❑ skin
❑ neurologic
❑ psychiatric
❑ heme/lymph/immune

Problem-focused = 1 element

Expanded problem-focused = 2–4 elements

Detailed = 5–7 elements

Comprehensive = 8 or more elements

EVALUATION AND MANAGEMENT AUDIT—MEDICAL DECISION MAKING

Number and types of problems established during the encounter, complexity of establishing a diagnosis, and management decisions that are made by the physician:

❑ minimal
❑ limited

❑ multiple
❑ extensive

Amount and complexity of data to be reviewed:

❑ minimal or none
❑ limited
❑ moderate
❑ extensive

Risk associated with the presenting problems, the diagnostic procedures, and the possible management options:

❑ minimal
❑ low
❑ moderate
❑ high

ASSESSMENT OF MEDICAL DECISION MAKING: From the lists above,
circle the appropriate levels on the grid below. If a column has at least two
circles, draw a line down that column to the type of medical decision making
on the bottom row. If no column has two circles, draw a line down the
column containing the second circle from the left.

Dx/mgmt	Minimal	Limited	Multiple	Extensive
Data	Min/none	Limited	Moderate	Extensive
Risk	Minimal	Low	Moderate	High
Decision making	Straight-forward	Low complex	Moderate complex	High complex

EVALUATION AND MANAGEMENT AUDIT—TOTAL

Circle below the levels of history, exam, and medical decision making
you selected above.

History	Problem-focused	Expanded prob-focus	Detailed	Comprehensive
Exam	Problem-focused	Expanded prob-focus	Detailed	Comprehensive
Decision making	Straight-forward	Low complex	Moderate complex	High complex

Using the definitions for levels of specific types of services, as found in the CPT manual, determine which level your documentation meets.

Two of the three elements (history, exam, decision making) must meet or exceed the defined level in order to assign that code in the following service categories:

- ❏ office, established patient
- ❏ inpatient, subsequent care
- ❏ inpatient, follow-up consult
- ❏ nursing facility, subsequent care
- ❏ boarding home, established patient
- ❏ home visit, established patient

Three of three elements must meet or exceed the stated requirements for all other services.

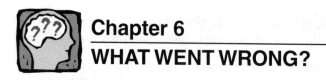

Chapter 6
WHAT WENT WRONG?

Your goal is to submit "clean claims." A key component is accurate documentation and coding. Clean claims are submitted in a timely manner, processed by the payer expeditiously, and are paid correctly, according to the payer's fee schedule, with no rejections or denials. The claims review process by third-party payers varies and is not infallible, so it is definitely worth assigning staff time to analyzing and resubmitting denied claims.

How do we make sure we have clean claims?

❏ Contact your major payers and determine what their time limits are for filing claims. Medicare is not typical in this regard, as it is among the most liberal. Some payers have filing limits as short as 30 to 45 days. Ask a staff member to make a chart showing these limits and post it on the wall in the billing area as a reminder.

❏ If you are using billing software, make sure it contains edits to at least prevent simple claims errors, such as invalid diagnosis and procedure codes, sex/diagnosis or sex/procedure conflicts, and/or age/diagnosis or age/procedure conflicts. Some software is capable of more sophisticated editing that may be worth the additional cost in the long run.

❏ You might consider using an electronic claims clearinghouse to file. These companies process claims for a fee, and most provide the same type of up-front editing that payers have.

How do we know why the claims were rejected or denied?

Learning to read payer remittance advice reports is mandatory if you are to revise and resubmit denied claims and obtain the reimbursement to which you are entitled. Payers each have their own cryptic abbreviations for why they have chosen not to pay you; payer manuals or newsletters usually contain a key to these codes.

Denial codes fall into several groups:

❏ Eligibility. Either the patient wasn't covered by this insurance on the date of service, or for some reason the payer can't find the patient in its files. Verify the claim information against the copy of the insurance card you keep in the patient's record and determine the problem.

❏ Invalid diagnosis codes. These either need more digits, were not valid on the date of service (*remember, the codes are updated annually*) or have a conflict with the patient's age, sex, etc.

❏ Invalid procedure codes. These codes were not valid on date of service or conflict, as above.

❏ Noncovered service. The patient's coverage with the insurer does not include this service. Common examples are: cosmetic surgery, in vitro fertilization, and routine physical exams with no documented complaint.

❏ Site of service conflict. This may arise if you visit a patient in the hospital whom you think is an inpatient, but he or she has been placed in observation status instead, or vice versa.

❏ Service not medically necessary. This means that the service you charged for is not considered medically necessary for the diagnosis reported. Not only are these denials becoming more prevalent as payers develop additional criteria for diagnostic testing, but your patient may also receive an explanation of benefits mentioning "not medically necessary," which may cause the patient to question your care. This category of denials is preventable if you and your staff keep up-to-date on the covered diagnoses. Remember the coding rules—if the diagnosis is not yet established, use the symptoms or signs prompting the testing. As always, make sure the documentation in the patient record matches your claims.

If you are, in fact, aware ahead of time that a service will be considered not medically necessary, you need to have the patient sign a beneficiary notice to this effect, acknowledging patient responsibility for the charges for that service. Without this signed notice, most payers will not allow you to bill the patient. The content and format of the notice may vary; contact your largest payers for samples.

❏ Duplicate service/bundled service/global service. These are all related to the global surgery package concept. Almost any time you bill more than one procedure on a date of service, you will probably need to use a modifier to explain why. If you are providing surgical services, modifiers will be needed for any services you provide during the global period to identify them as legitimately payable. Refer to Chapter 4, Translating the Record: Procedures, for detailed information on the use of modifiers.

If you and/or your staff do not understand why a claim is being denied, contact the payer. Make notes that you can keep with the patient's record for use in reviewing and possibly revising and resubmitting the claim or in discussing the denial with the patient.

How do we know which procedures require prior approval?

Most procedures performed in the office do not require prior approval by the payer. However, there are exceptions, and it is always better to call and ask first than be denied payment later for this reason. Many insurance cards have information on the back about referrals and approvals, along with telephone numbers. If your staff is told that no approval is necessary, this should be documented in the record, just like an approval, for future reference.

How do I appeal a claim?

Many payers offer telephone review/appeal. This is the first step if you think a minor error has caused your claim to be rejected. In some cases, the person you speak to will be able to correct the problem, and you won't have to resubmit the claim.

Government payers (Medicare, Medicaid, Champus) offer formal appeals processes with several levels of hearings, up to and including federal court. A surprisingly large percentage of Medicare denials are reversed at the first level of appeal, so it is worth trying.

To prepare for an appeal, you need to document why you think the denial was inappropriate. This may involve copies of records demonstrating medical necessity, along with a copy of the original claim, the denial letters, and a request for a hearing. If you find out that your local carrier has policies that do not agree with national policy, you may be able to appeal on those grounds.

Changes made to the national Correct Coding Initiative are not always implemented immediately, so be sure to check denials of this type to make sure they are in accordance with current policy. Your specialty societies often publish information about their successes in achieving changes in Correct Coding edits.

Warning!

A denial letter is *not* a signal to revise the patient's record to include a more "payable" diagnosis. If you truly forgot to document something at the time the service was provided, there is no problem with a properly documented late entry. This should be a rare occurrence. If you made a mistake and are denied payment as a result and are not successful in an appeal, look at it as a learning experience, an error to be avoided in the future.

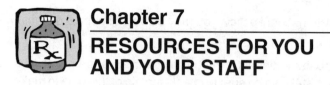

Chapter 7
RESOURCES FOR YOU AND YOUR STAFF

How can I get training for my staff?

The basis for coding competency starts with the fundamentals of medical terminology, anatomy, and physiology. If your staff has not studied these subjects, many local technical colleges or junior colleges offer courses. Medical terminology can be studied in the office through the use of programmed learning texts or audio/visual tapes. It is virtually impossible to learn correct coding principles without at least a basic understanding of medical terminology.

Are there certified coding professionals? How can my staff achieve these certifications?

CPC and CCS

Two national organizations offer certification in coding:

American Academy of Procedural Coders (AAPC)
145 W. Crystal Avenue
Salt Lake City, UT 84115
(800) 626-CODE
Certified Procedural Coder (CPC)
Certified Procedural Coder—Hospital (CPC-H)

American Health Information Management Association (AHIMA)
919 N. Michigan Avenue, Suite 1400
Chicago, IL 60611-1682
(800) 335-5535
Certified Coding Specialist (CCS)
Certified Coding Specialist-Physician Based (CCS-P)

All certifications are awarded upon successful completion of a national examination in the subject area. Contact these organizations directly for current requirements for examination.

ART and RRA

In addition, individuals certified by AHIMA as Accredited Record Technicians (ART) or Registered Record Administrators (RRA) have also passed exams including some elements of coding competency. AHIMA offers an independent study program, which, when combined with basic college courses, qualifies the individual to sit for the ART examination.

What are the basic resources my staff needs to code correctly?

❏ ICD-9-CM, CPT and HCPCS

At the very least, you must have current copies of ICD-9-CM CPT and HCPCS. It is not possible to skimp in this area of your budget. Using out-of-date coding books poses the risk of claims denials for use of discontinued codes. When you receive your new, updated books annually, take a look at the changes so you will be familiar with the latest terminology. Do not discard last year's books, however. A few payers, most notably workers' compensation carriers, are still using codes from a few years ago. Keeping five years' worth of books is probably a good idea, but put them away so they won't be used by mistake for current coding.

There are many sources for ordering versions of these publications. The AMA, AHIMA, and AAPC all carry publications of this type.

Other resources you will need are:

❏ Medical dictionary

❏ Medicare fee schedule database: tells which procedures can have various types of modifiers, what their type of service is (obtain from your Medicare carrier)

❏ *CPT Assistant.* Published by the AMA, this monthly newsletter contains useful articles and interpretive materials regarding CPT codes and their official definitions.

❏ *Coding Clinic.* Published by the Central Office on ICD-9-CM of the American Hospital Association, this is the official quarterly authority on ICD-9 diagnosis and procedure coding.

❏ References listed in Appendix C are also desirable.

❏ Many vendors also offer "encoders" for office use. While these are more convenient to use than the books, most require some knowledge of coding for correct use. The fact that you purchase an encoder does not mean you can hire an untrained person to use it and expect accurate coding.

How do I know how payers interpret codes?

Payer provider manuals and newsletters are one of the best sources for coding information. Citing a source from the payer itself is a very powerful tool in appealing a denied claim. Whether or not the payer notified providers that various services were not covered is also key in determining whether the provider "should have known" services would be denied. This can be an important element is assessment of whether a "pattern" of incorrect coding can be demonstrated.

My staff wants access to the Internet. Would this really be of much help in coding and documentation?

Absolutely! If you already use computers in your practice, adding a modem and Internet access can provide ready resources. The following websites are of interest:

AMA	www.ama-assn.org
AAPC	www.aapcnatl.org
AHIMA	www.ahima.org
NLM (National Library of Medicine)—literature searches on-line for free	www.nlm.nih.gov
HCFA (look up regulations, Office of Inspector General (OIG) reports, fraud and abuse information)	www.hcfa.gov
Managed links (links to managed care websites)	www.managedhealthlinks.com
National Center for Health Statistics (ICD-9-CM diagnosis codes)	www.cdc.gov/nchswww
Code of Federal Regulations	www.access.gpo.gov

Many professional societies, third-party payers, and federal and state government agencies also have websites with useful information.

After analyzing my billing and coding practices, I've decided I need professional help. How can I find a reliable consultant?

There are hundreds of consultants, and you are wise to look for reliability. The newspapers are full of ads soliciting individuals to "do medical billing at home in your spare time." Look for individuals with credentials, such as CPC, CCS, ART, or RRA, identifying that they are certified in this area. In order to get your money's worth, check with several sources: your colleagues, your professional society, your local or state medical or osteopathic association. In addition, the Medical Group Management Association (MGMA) is a national organization for medical practice managers, some of whom are consultants. They may be contacted at:

MGMA
104 Inverness Terrace East
Englewood, CO 80112-5306
(303) 799-1111

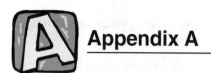 **Appendix A**

DIAGNOSTIC CODING AND REPORTING GUIDELINES FOR OUTPATIENT SERVICES (HOSPITAL BASED AND PHYSICIAN OFFICE) REVISED OCTOBER 1, 1995 (excerpts)

The terms encounter and visit are often used interchangeably in describing outpatient service contacts and, therefore, appear together in these guidelines without distinguishing one from the other.

Diagnoses often are not established at the time of the initial encounter/visit. It may take two or more visits before the diagnosis is confirmed.

A. The appropriate code or codes from 001.0 through V82.9 must be used to identify diagnoses, symptoms, conditions, problems, complaints, or other reasons for the encounter/visit.

B. For accurate reporting of ICD-9-CM diagnosis codes, the documentation should describe the patient's condition, using terminology that includes specific diagnoses as well as symptoms, problems, or reasons for the encounter. There are ICD-9-CM codes to describe all of these.

C. The selection of codes 001.0 through 999.9 will frequently be used to describe the reason for the encounter. These codes are from the section of ICD-9-CM for the classification of diseases and injuries (e.g., infectious and parasitic diseases; neoplasms; symptoms, signs, and ill-defined conditions, etc.)

D. Codes that describe symptoms and signs, as opposed to diagnoses, are acceptable for reporting purposes when an established diagnosis has not been diagnosed (confirmed) by the physician. Chapter 16 of ICD-9-CM, Symptoms, Signs, and Ill-defined Conditions (codes 780.799.9) contains many, but not all codes for symptoms.

E. ICD-9-CM provides codes to deal with encounters for circumstances other than a disease or injury. The Supplementary Classification of Factors Influencing Health Status and Contact with Health Services (V01.0–V82.9) is provided to deal with occasions when circumstances other than a disease or injury are recorded as diagnoses or problems.

F. ICD-9-CM is composed of codes with either 3, 4, or 5 digits. Codes with 3 digits are included in ICD-9-CM as the heading of a category of codes that may be further subdivided by the use of fourth and/or fifth digits that provide greater specificity. A three-digit code is to be used only if it is not further subdivided. Where fourth-digit subcategories and/or fifth-digit subclassifications are provided, they must be assigned. A code is invalid if it has not been coded to the full number of digits required for that code.

G. List first the ICD-9-CM code for the diagnosis, condition, problem, or other reason for encounter/visit shown in the medical record to be chiefly responsible for the services provided. List additional codes that describe any coexisting conditions.

H. Do not code diagnoses documented as "probable," "suspected," "questionable," "rule out," or "working diagnosis." Rather, code the condition(s) to the highest degree of certainty for that encounter/visit, such as symptoms, signs, abnormal test results, or other reason for the visit. Please note: This is contrary to the rules used by hospitals for coding the diagnoses of hospital inpatients.

I. Chronic diseases treated on an ongoing basis may be coded and reported as many times as the patient receives treatment and care for the condition(s).

J. Code all documented conditions that coexist at the time of the encounter/visit, and require or affect patient care treatment or management. Do not code conditions that were previously treated and no longer exist. However, history codes (V10-V19) may be used as secondary codes if the historical condition or family history has an impact on current care or influences treatment.

K. For patients receiving diagnostic services only during an encounter/visit, sequence first the diagnosis, condition, problem, or other reason for encounter/visit shown in the medical record to be chiefly responsible for the outpatient services provided during the encounter/visit. Codes for other diagnoses (e.g., chronic conditions) may be sequenced as additional diagnoses.

L. For patients receiving therapeutic services only during an encounter/ visit, sequence first the diagnosis, condition, problem, or other reason for encounter/visit shown in the medical record to be chiefly responsible for the outpatient services provided during the encounter/visit. Codes for other diagnosis (e.g., chronic conditions) may be sequenced as additional diagnoses. The only exception to this rule is that for patients receiving chemotherapy, radiation therapy, or rehabilitation, the appropriate V code for the service is listed first and the diagnosis or problem for which the service is being performed is listed second.

(The official guidelines contain no section M.)

N. For patient receiving preoperative evaluations only, sequence a code from category V72.8, Other specified examinations, to describe the preop consultations. Assign a code for the condition to describe the reason for the surgery as an additional diagnosis. Code also any findings related to the preop evaluation.

O. For ambulatory surgery, code the diagnosis for which the surgery was performed. If the postoperative diagnosis is known to be different from the preoperative diagnosis at the time the diagnosis is confirmed, select the postoperative diagnosis for coding, since it is the most definitive.

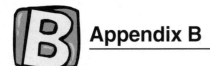 **Appendix B**

DATA ELEMENTS FOR DOCUMENTATION OF SERVICES

The following data elements should be considered for inclusion in your patient record forms and/or dictation outline. They are basic to documentation of services and justification for billing.

EVALUATION AND MANAGEMENT SERVICES

History

Chief Complaint (CC): concise statement describing the symptom, condition, diagnosis, physician-recommended return, or other factor that is the reason for the encounter, usually stated in the patient's own words.

History of Present Illness (HPI): a description of the development of the patient's present illness from the first sign and/or symptom, or from the previous encounter to the present. Elements of the HPI may include:

❏ location

❏ quality

❏ severity

❏ duration

❏ timing

❏ context

❏ modifying factors

❏ associated signs and symptoms

Review of Systems (ROS): an inventory of body systems obtained through a series of questions seeking to identify signs and/or symptoms that the patient may be experiencing or has experienced. The following systems are recognized:

❏ constitutional symptoms

- ❏ eyes

- ❏ ears, nose, mouth, throat

- ❏ cardiovascular

- ❏ respiratory

- ❏ gastrointestinal

- ❏ genitourinary

- ❏ musculoskeletal

- ❏ integumentary

- ❏ neurologic

- ❏ psychiatric

- ❏ endocrine

- ❏ hematologic/lymphatic

- ❏ allergic/immunologic

Past, Family, and/or Social History (PFSH):

- ❏ past history: patient's past experiences with illnesses, operations, injuries, and treatments

- ❏ family history: a review of medical events in the patient's family, including diseases that may be hereditary or place the patient at risk

- ❏ social history: an age-appropriate review of past and current activities

Examination

The items below are included in the general multisystem examination detailed by HCFA in its *Documentation Guidelines for Evaluation and Management Services*, May 1997:

Constitutional:

- ❏ measurement of any three of the following seven vital signs: sitting or standing blood pressure, supine blood pressure, pulse rate and regularity, respiration, temperature, height, weight

❑ general appearance of patient

Eye:

❑ inspection of conjunctivae and lids

❑ inspection of pupils and irises

❑ ophthalmoscopic exam of optic discs

ENT:

❑ external inspection of ears and nose

❑ otoscopic examination of external auditory canals and tympanic membranes

❑ assessment of hearing

❑ inspection of nasal mucosa, septum, and turbinates

❑ inspection of lips, teeth, and gums

❑ examination of oropharynx: oral mucosa, salivary glands, hard and soft palates, tongue, tonsils, and posterior pharynx

Neck:

❑ examination of neck

❑ examination of thyroid

Respiratory:

❑ assessment of respiratory effort

❑ percussion of chest

❑ palpation of chest

❑ auscultation of lungs

Cardiovascular:

❑ palpation of heart

❑ auscultation of heart with notation of abnormal sound and murmurs

❑ exam of carotid arteries

❑ exam of abdominal aorta

❏ exam of femoral arteries

❏ exam of pedal pulses

❏ exam of extremities for edema and/or varicosities

Chest (breasts):

❏ inspection of breasts

❏ palpation of breasts and axillae

Gastrointestinal:

❏ exam of abdomen with notation of presence of masses or tenderness

❏ exam of liver and spleen

❏ exam for presence or absence of hernia

❏ exam of anus, perineum, and rectum, including sphincter tone, presence of hemorrhoids, rectal masses

❏ obtain stool sample for occult blood, when indicated

Genitourinary:
(Female) Pelvic exam, including

❏ exam of external genitalia and vagina

❏ exam of urethra

❏ exam of bladder

❏ cervix

❏ uterus

❏ adnexa/parametria

(Male)

❏ exam of the scrotal contents

❏ exam of the penis

❏ digital rectal exam of prostate gland

Lymphatic:

❏ palpation of lymph nodes in two of the following areas:

- neck

- axillae

- groin

- other

Musculoskeletal:

❏ exam of gait and station

❏ inspection and/or palpation of digits and nails

❏ exam of joints, bones, and muscles of one or more of the following six areas: head and neck, R upper extremity, L upper extremity, R lower extremity, L lower extremity. Exam includes:

- inspection/palpation with notation of presence of any misalignment, asymmetry, crepitation, defects, tenderness, masses, or effusions

Skin:

❏ inspection of skin and subcutaneous tissue

❏ palpation of skin and subcutaneous tissue

Neurologic:

❏ test cranial nerves with notation of deficit

❏ exam of deep tendon reflexes

❏ exam of sensation

Psychiatric:

❏ description of judgment and insight

❏ mental status assessment, including:

- orientation to time, place, and person

- recent and remote memory

- mood and affect

In addition to the general multisystem exam, HCFA has also defined elements for 11 single-system exams. If you are a specialist, you need to obtain the specifications for these exams from your local Medicare carrier, or from the HCFA website at www.hcfa.gov/medicare/mcarpti.htm

Medical decision making:

Medical decision making refers to the complexity of establishing a diagnosis and/or selecting a management option, as measured by:

❏ the number of possible diagnoses and/or the number of management options that must be considered

❏ the amount and/or complexity of medical records, diagnostic tests, and/or other information that must be obtained, reviewed, and analyzed

❏ the risk of significant complications, morbidity, and/or mortality, as well as comorbidities, associated with the patient's presenting problems, the diagnostic procedures, and/or the possible management options.

Counseling and coordination of care

Physician discussion with the patient and/or family concerning:

❏ prognosis

❏ diagnostic results, impressions, recommended studies

❏ risks/benefits of treatment options

❏ instructions for treatment and/or follow-up

❏ importance of compliance with treatment plan

❏ risk factor reduction

❏ patient/family education

Time

❏ face-to-face time for outpatient services

❏ unit/floor time for inpatient services

PROCEDURES

In this context, "procedures" are all services other than E&M services. Thorough documentation of any procedure, whether office or operating room, includes:

❏ indications

❏ site

❏ laterality

❏ technique

CPT procedure descriptions are quite detailed. Familiarize yourself with those for the procedures you perform often, and use the official terminology in your documentation. Encourage your staff to talk with you if they are not clear about what procedures you performed.

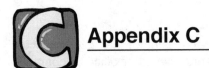 # Appendix C

BIBLIOGRAPHY

American Medical Association. (1998). *Physicians' current procedural terminology.* Chicago, IL.

Brown, F. (1998). *ICD-9-CM coding handbook.* Chicago, IL: American Hospital Publishing, Inc.

Health and Human Services Department, Centers for Disease Control and Prevention, Health Care Financing Administration. (1997). DHHS Publication PHS 97-1260. *International classification of diseases, ninth revision, clinical modification, sixth edition.* Washington, DC.

Kotoski, G., & Stegman, M. (1994). *Physician documentation for reimbursement.* Gaithersburg, MD: Aspen Publishers, Inc.

National Center for Health Statistics. "Diagnostic coding and reporting guidelines for outpatient services (hospital-based and physician office)." www.cdc.gov/nchswww/data/icdguide.pdf